COLON CANCER

CALMLY DEALING WITH ALL THE COMPLICATIONS OF COLON CANCER

DR. J. SIMON

Contents

INTRODUCTION

Colon cancer is one type of cancer that originates in the large intestine, which houses the colon and the rectum. Usually, it starts out as little polyps, which are collections of cells that are not malignant but have the potential to turn into cancer over time. The exact etiology of colon cancer is not always known, despite the fact that it is one of the most common diseases worldwide.

Colon cancer risk factors include advanced age, a family history of the condition, certain genetic disorders, inflammatory bowel diseases, a diet high in red or processed meats, obesity, smoking, and excessive alcohol consumption.

Some signs include altered bowel habits, blood in the stool, abdominal pain, unexplained weight loss, fatigue, or the feeling that the colon doesn't empty completely. Early detection through routine screenings, such colonoscopies, is crucial for effective therapy.

Treatment options for colon cancer can include surgery, chemotherapy, radiation therapy, targeted therapy, or a combination of these, depending on the stage and severity of the disease. People need to be aware of the risk factors, adopt preventative measures, and undergo the recommended screenings in order to detect colon cancer in its early and more treatable stages.

CHAPTER ONE

What Colorectal Cancer Means

Colon cancer is a type of cancer that originates in the colon, which is a portion of the large intestine. This kind of cancer often starts as abnormal growths called polyps, but it can eventually turn malignant. The colon and the rectum, which make up the large intestine, are both susceptible to cancer.

Unchecked cell growth in the colon's lining is the defining feature of colon cancer. This proliferation can result in tumors that infiltrate neighboring organs and, in more advanced stages, migrate to other parts of the body. Early identification is essential for effective treatment, which is why routine screenings like colonoscopies are recommended to identify and remove polyps before they turn into cancer.

Factors such as age, diet, genetics, family history, and specific medical conditions can increase the risk of colon cancer. Possible symptoms include altered bowel habits, blood in the stool, fatigue, weight loss, and other signs of digestive trouble.

When selecting a colon cancer treatment, the patient's overall condition, location, and stage are all crucial factors to take into account. Common therapies for the disease include radiation therapy, chemotherapy, surgery, and targeted therapy, sometimes in combination, to ensure optimal results.

The colon, often known as the big intestine, is a vital part of the digestive system. It is necessary for the body to eliminate waste, to create stool, and to absorb water and electrolytes from undigested meals. Let's now look at its composition and functions:

Anatomy

Cecum: The beginning of the colon, where the small and big intestines converge. The appendix is a small pouch that is located next to the cecum. Its function is unknown.

Ascending Colon: The right side of the abdomen is where the colon ascends.

Transverse Colon: It crosses the upper abdomen from right to left.

Colon Descending: The colon descends from the abdomen's left side.

The sigmoid colon refers to the S-shaped section that goes to the rectum.

Applications:

Water and electrolyte absorption: As undigested food passes through the colon, water and electrolytes are absorbed, transforming liquid chyme from the small intestine into more solid stools.

Formation of Feces: The colon contributes to the shape of waste material by absorbing water and compacting the remaining indigestible components.

Fecal Material Storage: The colon serves as a temporary holding area for feces until they are ready to be expelled.

Fermentation: A range of bacteria in the colon ferment undigested carbohydrates, producing gasses and some vitamins as a byproduct.

Elimination: When the feces reach the rectum, a muscular organ at the end of the colon, signals indicating the need for a bowel movement are sent to the brain. Subsequently, the anal sphincters relax, permitting the controlled release of waste via the anus.

Understanding the anatomy and physiology of the colon is essential to maintaining digestive health and preventing issues like diarrhea, constipation, and many colorectal illnesses, including colon cancer.

Different varieties of colon cancer can be classified based on a variety of factors, including the specific cells involved, the colon's location, and the cancer cells' microscopic appearance. Here are some common types of colon cancer:

Adenocarcinoma: The most prevalent type of colon cancer, accounting for around 95% of cases. Adenocarcinoma originates from the glandular cells that line the inside surface of the colon and rectum.

Mucinous Adenocarcinoma: The cancer cells of this type of adenocarcinoma include the slimy substance known as mucin. Mucinous adenocarcinoma typically has a distinctive appearance under a microscope.

Signet Ring Cell Carcinoma: This type of carcinoma has cells that, when viewed under a microscope, resemble a signet ring. These cells are distinct because they have a large, empty space in the center.

Serrated Adenocarcinoma: Sharp-edged colon polyps have the potential to become serrated adenocarcinomas under specific circumstances.

These tumors look like sawtoothed or serrated teeth when viewed under a microscope.

Carcinoid Tumors: Although they are uncommon, these tumors can develop in the colon. These cells are derived from neuroendocrine cells and develop slowly.

Gastrointestinal Stromal Tumors (GISTs): These tumors are most commonly found in the stomach and small intestine, although they can also grow in the colon. They start from the connective tissue cells in the wall of the gastrointestinal tract.

It is essential to comprehend how colon cancer is categorized in order to select the most effective course of treatment. The specific type, stage, and location of the cancer aid medical professionals in developing an effective treatment plan that is unique for each patient. Regular screenings and early discovery are crucial for identifying the kind of colon cancer and enabling timely treatment to begin.

Contributors to Hazards

There are many risk factors that contribute to the development of colon cancer. Knowing these things makes it easier for people to assess their risk and take precautions. Some common risk factors for colon cancer include the following:

Age: The risk of colon cancer rises with age, and those over 50 are more likely to receive a diagnosis. However, incidents can also occur in a person's younger years.

Family History: Individuals who have a family history of colorectal polyps or colon cancer are more vulnerable. Your risk increases dramatically if a parent, sibling, or child in your first degree of relationship also has the illness.

Inherited Genetic Syndromes: A number of genetic disorders, such as Lynch syndrome (hereditary nonpolyposis colorectal cancer, or HNPCC) and familial adenomatous polyposis (FAP), can significantly raise the risk of colon cancer.

Personal History of Colorectal Polyps or Cancer: Individuals with a history of colorectal polyps or cancer are at a higher risk of developing them again.

IBD stands for inflammatory bowel diseases. Crohn's disease and ulcerative colitis are two chronic inflammatory bowel diseases that have been related to a higher risk of colon cancer.

Nutritional Factors: Eating a diet heavy in red and processed meats and low in fiber increases your chance of developing colon cancer. Diets rich in fruits, vegetables, and whole grains are associated with a lower risk.

Lack of Exercise: Studies have linked a sedentary lifestyle and infrequent exercise to an increased risk of colon cancer.

Obesity: Being overweight or obese raises the risk of colon cancer, particularly in men.

Smoking: Studies have indicated that smoking raises the risk of both colon and other cancers.

Alcohol use: Excessive alcohol use has been associated with a heightened risk of colon cancer.

Type 2 Diabetes: People with type 2 diabetes have an increased risk of colon cancer.

It's important to keep in mind that while some risk factors may increase your likelihood of developing colon cancer, the illness does not always follow. However, even without these risk factors are still susceptible to colon cancer. Early detection and successful treatment of colon cancer depend on a healthy lifestyle, routine testing, and awareness of potential signs.

Signs and Suggestions

It is crucial to recognize the warning signs and symptoms of colon cancer in order to receive timely medical attention and diagnose the disease early. Some common signs and symptoms of colon cancer include the following:

Constipation, diarrhea, or a change in the consistency of the stool are examples of persistent changes in bowel habits that may indicate colon cancer.

Blood in the Stool: Rectal bleeding or blood in the stool may be a severe sign that colon cancer is growing. Because blood may be seen on the feces, it may seem dark or black.

Constant abdominal pain, discomfort, or cramping should be treated, especially if it is not connected to any other known medical conditions.

Unexplained Weight reduction: If no dietary, exercise, or other changes can account for the unintentional weight reduction, it may be due to colon cancer.

Fatigue: Severe weakness or exhaustion that does not improve with resting could indicate several medical conditions, including colon cancer.

Incomplete Bowels Emptying: You might have a tumor or obstruction in your colon if you feel that your bowel motions do not empty completely beyond that point.

Iron Deficiency Anemia: This condition can be brought on by even minor persistent gastrointestinal bleeding. Pale skin, tiredness, or weakness could be the signs.

Narrow Stools: Thin or pencil-shaped stool may be a sign of blockage or constriction in the colon.

It's important to keep in mind that same symptoms can also be associated with benign issues or other gastrointestinal ailments. In the event that any of these symptoms persist for more than a few days or are accompanied by other concerning symptoms, it is recommended that you seek emergency medical attention. Routine testing like colonoscopies are necessary for early detection of colon cancer in order to reduce its effects and increase the likelihood of a positive outcome.

Recognizing and Avoiding

In order to detect cancer in its early stages, when treatment options are more favorable, or to identify and remove precancerous polyps, colon cancer screening is crucial for early detection. Some common methods for early detection and screening for colon cancer include the following:

Colonoscopies are the most effective method of screening for colon cancer. During a colonoscopy, a flexible tube with a camera is inserted into the colon to observe the whole length of the large intestine. If polyps are found during the procedure, they can be removed to reduce the chance that cancer will become apparent.

The Fecal Occult Blood Test (FOBT) detects blood clots in the stool, which could be a sign of colon cancer or precancerous polyps. You can complete this non-invasive test at home using the kit your doctor will give you.

Fecal Immunochemical Test (FIT): Similar to FOBT, FIT does not require any dietary restrictions before to the test and is more specific to human blood. Still, it finds blood in the stool.

Stool DNA Test: This test looks for particular DNA changes in cells secreted into the stool by polyps or colon cancer. It can be done at home and is less invasive than a colonoscopy.

Virtual Colonoscopy (CT Colonography): Using computed tomography (CT) scans, this imaging technique produces finely detailed images of the colon. Although it may not require anesthesia like a traditional colonoscopy, it may still need bowel preparation.

Flexible Sigmoidoscopy: In this technique, the rectum and lower portion of the colon are examined using a flexible sigmoidoscope. It cannot reach as far as a colonoscopy, but it can detect abnormalities in the lower portion of the colon.

Recommendations for screening techniques and frequency may vary depending on characteristics such as age, personal and family medical history, and risk factors. It is essential that people speak with their healthcare provider to determine which screening strategy is most appropriate for their unique situation.

Regular screenings are required because, even in otherwise healthy individuals, colon cancer can grow in its early stages without exhibiting any symptoms. Early detection significantly increases the chance that a patient with colon cancer will receive a successful therapy and experience improved outcomes.

Recognition

The diagnosis of colon cancer involves a variety of tests and examinations to determine the disease's presence, stage, and appropriate course of therapy. A summary of the process for diagnosing colon cancer is given below:

Medical History and Physical Examination:

The patient's past medical history is enquired about by healthcare experts, together with any symptoms the patient may have experienced and any family history of cancer.

A physical examination of the rectum and the lower part of the colon may be performed, maybe using a digital rectal exam.

Blood Tests:

Two blood tests that can be used to assess overall health and search for signs of anemia or abnormal liver function are complete blood counts (CBCs) and blood chemistry panels.

Imaging Tests:

A colonoscopy is a vital tool for identifying colon cancer. A flexible tube with a camera is inserted into the colon to examine the whole length of the large intestine. Throughout the procedure, biopsies could be obtained for extra investigation.

Virtual colonoscopy, also known as CT colonography, is an imaging procedure that uses CT scans to provide exact images of the colon, which helps identify any abnormalities more easily.

To assess the degree of the cancer and determine whether it has spread to any other organs or tissues, CT scans of the abdomen and pelvis can be performed.

MRI: Magnetic resonance imaging (MRI) can be used to get detailed images of the colon and its surrounds.

If abnormal tissue or polyps are discovered during a colonoscopy, a biopsy is performed. Tissue samples can be examined under a microscope to determine the kind and presence of cancer by sending them to a pathology lab.

Location:

Once the diagnosis has been confirmed, the cancer is staged to determine its extent and spread. Staging has a role in guiding treatment decisions. For staging, other imaging tests like CT or PET scans can be required.

Genetic Analysis:

Some people may decide to undergo genetic testing if there is a family history of colon cancer in order to identify specific genetic abnormalities associated with an increased risk of the disease.

The diagnosis of colon cancer is a multidisciplinary procedure that includes radiologists, pathologists, and medical professionals. To improve prognoses and develop an effective treatment plan, individuals with colon cancer require early identification and a clear diagnosis.

Phase and Prospects

Determining the severity and extent of colon cancer, making treatment decisions, and evaluating the disease's prognosis all depend on knowing the stage of the disease. The most popular staging method for colon cancer is the

TNM method, which takes into account three crucial factors.

T (Tumor): Represents the size of the primary tumor.

TX: There is no evidence of the initial tumor.

T0: There is no visible primary tumor.

T1, T2, T3, T4: The size and/or extent of the initial tumor steadily expanding.

N (Nodes): Indicates whether the cancer has impacted nearby lymph nodes.

NX: Regional lymph nodes cannot be evaluated.

N0: No local lymph nodes are involved.

N1, N2: The number of lymph nodes involved and their level of involvement; N2 indicates a more extensive spread.

M (metastasis): Indicates if the malignancy has spread to distant organs or tissues.

M0: There are no distant metastases.

M1: Distant metastases are present.

The combined T, N, and M variables can determine a colon cancer's stage, which can range from 0 (early stage) to IV (advanced stage). The higher the stage, the more advanced the cancer.

Colon cancer stages:

Stage0: Only the inner lining of the colon is affected; no deeper layers are infiltrated.

Stage I: Not present in the muscular layer or barely slightly present.

Stage II: Incurs into or passes through the muscular layer, but does not impact nearby lymph nodes.

Stage III: Impacts surrounding lymph nodes and the colon's outer layers.

Stage IV: The cancer has spread to other organs or tissues.

CHAPTER TWO

Prediction:

The expected course and outcome of the sickness are described by the word "prognosis". The location of the tumor, the patient's overall health, the stage of diagnosis, and the efficacy of the treatment plan are a few factors that influence the prognosis for colon cancer. In general:

The prognosis is usually positive and there is a higher likelihood of long-term survival in the early stages (Stages I and II).

Stage III (intermediate stage): The prognosis is still favorable with the appropriate treatment, including chemotherapy and surgery.

Stage IV: The outlook is worse because the cancer has spread to other organs. The purpose of therapy is to control symptoms and extend life.

Early detection, regular screenings, and advancements in therapy have all contributed to a better overall prognosis for colon cancer patients. Since each patient reacts to treatment differently, ongoing monitoring and follow-up care are essential for managing the condition and any possible recurrence.

Treatment Options

Numerous factors, including the patient's overall health and the stage and location of the cancer, influence the treatment plan for colon cancer. Commonly available treatments for colon cancer include:

Surgery:

Polypectomy: A little polyp is removed during a colonoscopy.

Colectomy: The surgical removal of the affected portion of the colon. Another alternative would be to remove any neighboring lymph nodes.

Dissection of the Lymph Nodes: removing neighboring lymph nodes to search for signs of malignant development.

Chemotherapy:

medicine intended to stop the growth of cancer cells or to completely eradicate them. For advanced stages, it can be used as the primary course of treatment, as a neoadjuvant before to surgery, or as an adjuvant following surgery.

Radiation Therapy:

High-energy lasers are used to target and destroy cancer cells. It is not commonly used for early-stage colon cancer, however it may be administered during therapy for rectal cancer.

Personalized Health Care:

medications that particularly target chemicals linked to the onset of cancer. These drugs may be used in addition to chemotherapy for advanced stages.

Immunotherapy:

improving the ability of the immune system to recognize and destroy malignant cells. Although it is more commonly used to treat other cancers, research is currently being done to investigate its potential for treating colon cancer.

Clinical Assessments:

taking part in clinical studies that assess new treatments or combinations of treatments. This decision is often considered in situations that are intricate or recurrent.

Hospice Medical Services:

focuses on managing symptoms and improving quality of life for patients with advanced or inoperable colon cancer. It helps with discomfort management and enhances overall wellness even if it does not attempt to treat the ailment.

The treatment decision is determined by a number of factors, including the patient's overall health, the tumor's location and stage, and the presence of specific genetic abnormalities. To develop treatment plans, medical specialists such as radiologists, surgeons, oncologists, and others often collaborate in a multidisciplinary manner.

It is imperative that patients discuss treatment options, potential adverse effects, and expected outcomes with their healthcare team. To monitor the efficacy of treatment, manage side effects, and address any potential recurrence of colon cancer, routine follow-up care is essential. Patients with colon cancer now have a far better prognosis thanks to advances in early detection and therapy.

Nutritional support

For patients undergoing treatment for colon cancer, supportive nutrition is critical to their overall health. A nutritious diet strengthens the immune system, encourages recovery, and reduces side effects from medication. Some general dietary recommendations for support during and after colon cancer treatment are as follows:

Maintain a Balanced Diet:

Make eating a diet rich in fruits, vegetables, whole grains, and lean meats a priority.

Add a variety of colorful fruits and vegetables to ensure a broad range of nutrients.

Adequate Consumption of Protein:

Tissue healing and immune response require protein. Include sources of lean protein such as tofu, beans, chicken, and fish.

Healthy Fats:

Include high-fat foods such as avocados, nuts, seeds, and olive oil in your diet.

Consuming lots of water

Especially before, during, and after therapy, make sure you consume lots of water. Drinking enough water helps manage side effects like diarrhea and improves overall health.

Fiber Intake:

Increase your intake of fiber gradually, especially if you are experiencing digestive issues or are undergoing surgery. Foods high in fiber include fruits, vegetables, and whole grains.

Small, Frequent Meals:

Smaller, more frequent meals will aid with digestion and minimize discomfort or nausea.

Limit processed and red meats:

Consuming red and processed meats should be avoided since they may increase the risk of colon cancer.

Calcium with vitamin D:

One has to get adequate calcium and vitamin D for healthy bones, especially if dairy products are off limits due to pharmaceutical side effects.

Extras as Needed:

Depending on the needs of each patient, medical specialists may provide nutritional smoothies, vitamins, or minerals as supplements.

Consult a Qualified Nutritionist:

A licensed dietician with experience in cancer can provide tailored guidance based on specific treatment regimens, side effects, and nutritional needs.

Both before and after therapy, patients may experience side effects that impair their appetite, such as nausea, taste changes, or difficulty swallowing. You should speak with your healthcare professionals about any nutritional concerns you may have and seek advice from a licensed nutritionist.

Seek medical guidance before making significant dietary changes or adding supplements. This is due to the fact that every patient has different nutritional needs depending on their specific situation throughout colon cancer treatment.

Survival and Reconstruction

When referring to colon cancer, "survivorship" is the period of time that follows the end of initial therapy when patients transition from active treatment to ongoing care, monitoring, and maintenance of their health. Important aspects of colon cancer survivability and post-treatment care include the following:

Verify Appointments Again:

Making regular follow-up appointments with the oncologist is essential to monitoring any new developments or recurrence indicators.

Imaging and Check-Ups:

To keep an eye out for any changes or recurrences in the colon, it may be necessary to schedule regular imaging tests, such as colonoscopies or CT scans.

Blood Tests:

Blood tests can be used to monitor carcinoembryonic antigen (CEA) levels as a potential indicator of cancer recurrence.

Discussing Adverse Reactions and Delayed Reactions:

Survivorship care includes managing and treating any residual side effects from treatment. It could be required for this to collaborate with other medical professionals such as dietitians, physiotherapists, or mental health specialists.

Emotional and Psychosocial Support:

A stable emotional existence is necessary for survival. People often experience anxiety, despair, and recurrent feelings of dread. Resources for therapy, support groups, and mental health issues can be beneficial.

Encouraging a healthy lifestyle:

Promoting a healthy lifestyle that forgoes tobacco and excessive alcohol use, engages in regular exercise, and eats a balanced food is essential to survival.

Watching for recurrent malignancies:

Those who have survived colon cancer may be at a higher risk of developing new primary cancers. When it comes to monitoring and preventive actions, healthcare providers may be contacted.

Genetic Advice:

Those with a genetic predisposition to colon cancer or a family history of the disease may benefit from ongoing genetic counseling.

Keeping One's Health:

Scheduling routine medical checks, vaccinations, and screenings for other disorders is essential for overall health.

Instructions for Patients:

Ongoing education regarding warning signs and symptoms of recurrence, potential side effects, and the importance of self-care empowers survivors to actively participate in their own health.

A survivor and the oncology team often collaborate to construct survivorship care plans, which offer a timetable for ongoing support and treatment. It is imperative that survivors communicate any concerns, symptoms, or changes in their health to medical experts in an open and honest manner.

The goal of survivorship a dynamic and singular journey is to assist individuals in moving forward from their colon cancer experience with a healthy and meaningful life. Regular follow-up care is essential for preserving long-term wellbeing, keeping an eye on health, and responding quickly to any issues that arise.

Prevention and Lifestyle Techniques

By adopting preventive measures and living a healthy lifestyle, one can significantly reduce the risk of colon cancer. Here are some recommendations for lifestyle and prevention:

Maintain a Nutritious Diet:

Eat a diet rich in whole grains, lean proteins, fruits, and vegetables, as well as balance.

Because red and processed meats have been associated with an increased risk of colon cancer, they should be consumed in moderation.

Maintain Your Exercise:

Engage in regular exercise, such as jogging, cycling, brisk walking, or other high-intensity sports.

Aim for 150 minutes or more per week of moderate-to-intense exercise.

Maintain an Appropriate Weight:

An increased risk of colon cancer has been associated with obesity. Combine a nutritious diet with frequent exercise to reach your goal weight.

Limit Your Alcohol Consumption:

Limit your alcohol intake because too much of it has been linked to a higher risk of colon cancer.

Quit Smoking:

Colon cancer is among the many malignancies that smoking has been connected to. There are many health advantages to giving up smoking.

Frequent Exams:

To identify cancer at an early stage or to detect and remove precancerous polyps, adhere to recommended screening guidelines, such as colonoscopies.

Understand Your Lineage:

Know the medical history of your family, particularly with regard to colon cancer. People with a family history might require screenings more frequently or earlier.

Handle Long-Term Illnesses:

Diabetes and other chronic illnesses should be managed because they raise the risk of colon cancer.

Increase Fiber Intake:

Include fiber-rich foods in your diet, such as whole grains, fruits, and vegetables. Fiber may help promote regular bowel movements and reduce the risk of colon cancer.

Maintain Hydration:

Adequate hydration is essential for overall health and may also contribute to a healthy digestive system.

Consider Aspirin or NSAIDs:

In certain cases, aspirin or nonsteroidal anti-inflammatory drugs (NSAIDs) may be recommended for individuals at high risk of colon cancer. However, this should be discussed with a healthcare professional, as these medications have potential risks.

CHAPTER THREE

Limit Processed Foods:

Reduce the intake of processed and highly refined foods, as they may contribute to an increased risk of colon cancer.

Remember that individual risk factors vary, and it's crucial to consult with healthcare professionals for personalized advice based on your health history and circumstances. Making informed lifestyle choices and adopting preventive strategies can contribute to a reduced risk of developing colon cancer and promote overall well-being.

The emotional and psychological impact of colon cancer can be profound, affecting both individuals diagnosed with the disease and their loved ones. Here are some common emotional and psychological aspects associated with colon cancer:

Fear and Anxiety:

The diagnosis of cancer often brings feelings of fear and anxiety about the future, treatment, and potential outcomes.

Depression:

Dealing with a serious illness like colon cancer can lead to feelings of sadness and depression.

Coping with the physical and emotional challenges of treatment may contribute to emotional distress.

Uncertainty and Ambiguity:

The uncertainty surrounding the course of treatment, potential side effects, and the overall prognosis can create feelings of ambiguity and distress.

Changes in Body Image:

Surgical procedures, ostomies, or changes in physical appearance due to treatment may impact body image, self-esteem, and confidence.

Grief and Loss:

Coping with the loss of normalcy, lifestyle changes, and the impact on relationships may lead to feelings of grief.

Social Isolation:

Some individuals may withdraw from social activities or feel isolated as they navigate the challenges of cancer treatment.

Impact on Relationships:

The emotional toll of cancer can strain relationships with family, friends, and partners. Open communication is crucial for mutual support.

Role Changes:

Individuals may experience changes in their roles and responsibilities, such as shifts in employment, caregiving dynamics, or financial concerns.

Coping with Treatment Side Effects:

Dealing with the physical side effects of treatment, such as fatigue, nausea, and pain, can contribute to emotional distress.

Post-Treatment Adjustment:

The transition from active treatment to survivorship may bring a mix of emotions, including relief, gratitude, and adjustment to a "new normal."

Impact on Mental Health:

Individuals with a history of mental health issues may find that the stress of a cancer diagnosis exacerbates their emotional well-being.

It's essential for individuals facing colon cancer to seek emotional support and resources to address these challenges. Strategies for coping may include:

Counseling and Psychotherapy: Professional counseling can provide a safe space to express emotions, explore coping strategies, and navigate the psychological impact of cancer.

Support Groups: Connecting with others who have experienced or are experiencing similar challenges can offer a sense of community and understanding.

Mind-Body Practices: Techniques such as mindfulness, meditation, and yoga may help manage stress and improve emotional well-being.

Open Communication: Honest and open communication with healthcare providers, loved ones, and support networks is crucial for addressing emotional needs.

Self-Care: Prioritizing self-care activities, hobbies, and activities that bring joy and relaxation can contribute to emotional well-being.

It's important for individuals and their loved ones to recognize the emotional impact of colon cancer and seek appropriate support. Healthcare providers, social workers, and mental health professionals can play key roles in helping individuals navigate the emotional challenges associated with the diagnosis and treatment of colon cancer.

CONCLUSION

colon cancer is a significant health concern with wide-ranging implications for individuals and their loved ones. Early detection through regular screenings, awareness of risk factors, and a healthy lifestyle are critical in preventing and managing this disease.

The journey through colon cancer involves various aspects, from the initial diagnosis and treatment to survivorship. Advances in medical research and treatment options have improved outcomes, allowing individuals to lead fulfilling lives beyond their cancer experience.

The emotional and psychological impact of colon cancer cannot be overlooked. Fear, uncertainty, and changes in body image can take a toll on mental health. Seeking emotional support, whether through counseling, support groups, or open communication with healthcare providers and loved ones, is essential for coping with the challenges that arise.

As we continue to deepen our understanding of colon cancer and refine treatment approaches, it's crucial to emphasize the importance of holistic care. This includes addressing physical, emotional, and psychological well-being, supporting individuals through their entire cancer journey, and promoting a sense of resilience and hope.

Ultimately, early detection, advancements in treatment, and ongoing research offer hope in the fight against colon cancer. By fostering awareness, encouraging preventive measures, and providing comprehensive support, we can work towards a future where the impact of colon cancer is minimized, and individuals can lead healthier lives.

THE END